Aromatherapy

Essential Aromatherapy and Oil Guide for Health, Happiness and Stress Relief

Anti-Cellulite Balm

Belly Busting massage oil

Aromatherapy anti stress massage oil

Aromatherapy Bath Salt

CONCLUSION

Introduction

Thank you for purchasing the book, '*Aromatherapy: Essential Aromatherapy and Oil Guide for health, Happiness and Stress Relief*'.

When it comes to grooming, people all across the world make a keen effort of the same. In the earlier times, grooming did not involve the number of cosmetics that are used by people now. These cosmetics are loaded with numerous chemicals that will make you question whether or not they actually help in making a person look prettier. The answer to this question is no and this is something that has been accepted by people all across the world. Though we know that these cosmetics are not good for our health, we tend to purchase them every month because we are unaware of the natural products that exist.

It is the same dilemma that we face when we are looking for ways to stay healthy and fit. We have trusted the numerous pills that are in the market on the pretext that they are the best way to heal ourselves. Little do we know that there is an option to use natural products that would leave us in better health and without any side effects?

There is one method that has held a key position when it comes to healing and grooming in the ancient times and this method goes by the name aromatherapy. If you are a beginner and are unaware of what aromatherapy is all about, you do not have to worry since this book will guide you through it all. This book contains all the vital information that you will need to know about aromatherapy and the usage of essential oils for the same.

The first few chapters of the book leave you with the basic information about aromatherapy that is essential for you to know. You have also been given the list of essential oils that you could use to keep yourself healthy and happy!

Thank you for purchasing this book. I truly hope you find it interesting.

Chapter 1: About Aromatherapy

This chapter covers the basic details about aromatherapy. You will find this information helpful when it comes to identifying the right oils that you will need to use in order to calm yourself down or to keep yourself happy. You will also find that these oils help you keep yourself and your life beautiful!

What is aromatherapy?

This is the first question that may have crossed your mind. You may have begun to wonder what exactly it is and how it helps you relieve yourself of stress and also helps in keeping you healthy. Aromatherapy is just that – you will find a way to live in a healthy way by using essential oils. When I am talking about health I mean both physical and mental health. The technique of using aromatherapy is not something that was developed recently. The practice has resurfaced in the last few years in order to ensure that people live happily and lead a healthy lifestyle.

Aromatherapy and its history

As mentioned above, aromatherapy is not a new age technique that has been developed to aid the health of human beings. It is in fact a practice that has existed centuries ago! It was when Jesus Christ was born that aromatherapy was first used by the people. This would lead to the belief that the practice of aromatherapy does date back to over 4000 years. There are numerous civilizations that have used the oils from different plants in order to provide medicine for their injured or sick.

There are deep roots for aromatherapy in India that has been mentioned explicitly in the writings of the healers in the ancient era. It was during this period that the Indians had experimented with 700 plants and identified their medicinal properties. They named these oils essential oils since these are required to maintain good health. These oils were used for aromatherapy in Ayurveda that is a traditional form of Indian medicine. The aromatherapy was used to give the patients full body massages with the essential oils. These massages then gained huge popularity in the West!

When the uses of these oils spread to different countries, the Chinese tried to use these oils to cure their people of certain illnesses. A certain Chinese pharmacist, Shen Nung had written a book enlisting all the herbs that could be used for their medicinal properties. This book has the properties of 400 such herbs and plants. It was during the same period that the Egyptians also started to use the essential oils. They had started to excel in the extraction of essential oils which helped them cure illnesses and also pay homage to the Gods they worshipped. They would burn the incense or fragrance sticks in front of God in order to show respect. They did a little more than this with the usage of essential oils for aromatherapy.

The Egyptians began to use the oils from the Chamomile and the Galbanum plants in order to clean the bodies of their Pharaohs. They had to clean their bodies before they embalmed them in their resting place. The resting place of the Pharaoh has Cinnamon, Cassia and Myrrh oils in order to impart greater fragrance. To ensure that the Pharaohs smelled their best before they were embalmed, the Egyptians used to dip the wrapping cloth in oils of juniper, cedarwood, myrrh and cinnamon. They had realized that these oils helped in preserving the body of the Pharaoh to an extent once they were embalmed. There were other Egyptians, who were wealthy, who purchased essential oils to use them to care for their skin. The Greeks and the Romans were not that far behind when it came to the use of essential oils. They had mastered the use of aromatherapy and begin to use the essential oils as a part of their medicines.

It is only in the past decade that people have realized that aromatherapy is of great importance. There is a possibility that you are wondering what it is that aromatherapy is all about. You would have come across many salons and spas that have a lot of massages which use the aroma of the essential oils, aromatherapy, in order to relieve any stress or to simply relieve certain parts of their body. But why would I be asking you to try aromatherapy?

The why behind aromatherapy?

There are numerous benefits of aromatherapy that have been covered in detail in the next chapter. But, before I compel you to go on further, I have enlisted a few benefits that are the best you can obtain when you use aromatherapy.

Stress and Pain Relief

In today's fast paced world, people are always overburdened with the different roles they have to perform on a regular basis. When you use aromatherapy, you will be able to find a way to push this stress and anxiety out of your head. You will find yourself as calm as a leaf. You had read earlier that Ayurveda had used aromatherapy to cure patients. This is because the massages that used essential oils helped in easing various types of pain.

Induces Sleep

Another brilliant benefit of Aromatherapy is to overcome insomnia that is caused due to excessive stress and anxiety. You could use aromatherapy to fall asleep on time to ensure that you do not wake up with droopy eyes.

Skin Care

Essential oils are excellent at treating your skin. You will find that you are able to cure your skin of any acne or any other form of a rash by using certain essential oils. The oils help in smoothening and moisturizing your skin.

Improving Digestive capacity and Immunity

There are several essential oils used in aromatherapy that always have a positive effect on the functioning of our digestive system. You will find certain oils listed in the last chapter which will help you understand which oil you can use to aid digestion. The oils help in giving your immune system the boost that it needs in order to function well.

Hair Care

To care for your hair becomes easier when you begin to use essential oils. You will find that you can treat your hair naturally for all the problems you claim that you may have. You will find that your hair begins to grow better than it used to.

Antibacterial and Antifungal properties

Almost every essential oil has an antibacterial or an antifungal property that help in curing any infection or any other abrasions that you may have. These oils are natural and contain no chemicals that may cause any side effects to you.

These are certain key benefits which would need to be remembered when you are beginning to practice aromatherapy. There are other benefits that have been mentioned in detail in the next chapter.

Essential Oils and what are they?

You may have gathered a decent idea on what aromatherapy is and how you can use it. But, before I go into the details about the different oils to use, let me explain to you what essential oils are. These oils are certain liquids that have been extracted by different processes from various parts of plants. These oils have various properties that can be utilized by you in order to heal yourself. But, these oils are very different from the regular oils that you use.

Viscosity

The essential oils that you often come across are not as viscous as the regular oils that you use at home. They do not stick to your skin the way the regular oils do either.

Aroma

The oils have a lovely smell that is unique to them. These smells are the ones that make aromatherapy a success since they instill a sense of calm when inhaled.

Source

The essential oils are often those that are extracted from different parts of the plant while the regular oils are often extracted from the seeds of the plants.

The above-mentioned differences are only a few of what may be a million differences between essential and regular oils. The most common essential oils that are found are tea tree oil, rose oil, geranium oil, sandalwood oil, lavender oil and many more.

The main thing to remember is that there are certain oils, called carrier oils that are required to ensure that the essential oils mix well. The oils that are used more often than others are – olive oil, walnut oil, jojoba oil and almond oil.

Chapter 2: Why Use Essential Oils?

In the previous chapter you have been told about what aromatherapy is and a few of your questions about aromatherapy have been answered. There is a possibility that you still are not convinced about using aromatherapy, but this chapter should shove all your doubts away. You will be able to understand why essential oils are used for aromatherapy and not regular oils.

Zero Side effects

The essential oils are all natural products and have been extracted without the usage of any chemicals as mentioned in the next chapter of the book. It is because of this fact that these oils almost never have any side effects. This is one of the main reasons behind why it is essential that you use aromatherapy to keep you happy! All of us know that there is a chance of having some side effect or the possibility of having an over dose when you consume pharmaceutical drugs. These issues are all non – existent when you consider essential oils. The latter parts of the book will also help you boost your immune system and also improve your health rapidly. But, before all this, you will have to learn how to use essential oils which has been mentioned in the next chapter.

Detox

The food that you have been consuming over the years is the cause of the accumulation of numerous toxins in your body. These toxins could also be in your body due to the fact that you are constantly out in the open where there is a lot of pollution.

These toxins have a terrible effect on your immune system leaving you weak and unhealthy. If they are not removed fast enough, you will be leading yourself onto a path that is self – destructive. You could use certain essential oils that are antioxidants to help you rid your body of the many toxins in it.

Market Availability

Most drugs can only be purchased in the market only from a few chemists if you have a prescription from your doctor. The best fact about essential oils is that they can be found in any place! You could walk to the dollar store near your house or to the supermarket and you would find a wide range of essential oils in the racks at the stores! You will only have to add a few essential oils to your grocery list that would remind you to purchase them! If you are someone who does not want to always purchase essential oils, you have the option to plant the herbs or the plants in your backyard and extract the oils from them! The next chapter leaves you with a do – it – yourself method that would help you extract the oil that you want.

Safe

Your doctor would have told you that you would need to follow a certain diet when it comes to the consumption of a few of the pharmaceutical drugs. If you do not meet the conditions that have been stipulated, you would be harming yourself in a way you would never have been able to imagine. The essential oils are nothing like this! As mentioned earlier, there are no side effects to the essential oils that would give you the confidence that you would never have to worry about the side effects! But, you will need to be careful that you do not use too much of the essential oil.

Multiple Benefits

The multiple pharmaceutical drugs that have been produced only cater to one sort of illness or issue. You will find that you can never use the same drug for a different use! If you have to take good care of yourself, you will need to consume multiple pills that would be a bad idea!

If you are using essential oils, you will find that you gain multiple benefits from the oil! You will find that the oils help you cure multiple health issues – both physical and mental – if you are using essential oils. For instance, sandalwood oil helps in weight reduction and in relieving you of any stress. Another fact to remember is that you could use any proportion of the essential oil if you know where to use it! This cannot be said about the pharmaceutical drugs. You will find that you look young and carefree when you begin to use the essential oils and also keep yourself from causing yourself any harm.

Cheap and readily available

Pharmaceutical drugs have always been very expensive. They are always priced in a way that would give the manufacturers and the pharmacists a large profit! These drugs have never been priced in a way that would give every person the chance to purchase the drug. You will find that these drugs are expensive and a lot of savings would be used up to purchase these drugs. You could find such an example in almost every person all across Africa. This is because of the fact that the citizens of Africa have little or no exposure at all and will find it difficult to differentiate between the different drugs.

If you have decided to make use of the pharmaceutical drugs, you will have to ensure that you identify the right store in order to purchase the drug. But, if you are looking at cheaper methods of treatment, you will need to try aromatherapy. This is because of the fact that the essential oils used for the therapy are found in the market abundantly. The greatest part is that these oils can be made in your very own backyard! You will find that you can save enough money when it comes to using essential oils since they are cost effective.

Stress Reliever

People in this world have never been laid back and have always been under extreme levels of stress and pressure. This stress has become a part of the family! There are numerous factors that would be the cause of stress but you may have been overlooking these factors in order to move on in your life. This ultimately leads to many health issues!

Stress has been found to affect your body in adverse ways by first targeting your organs. Since it is this talented, it is essential that you keep an eye out for the amount of stress you have in order to keep yourself healthy. You will find most people around you consuming multiple pills to keep the stress at bay. What they tend to forget is that these pills have adverse effects which will only surface at a later point in life. Some people have used sleeping pills in order to fall asleep in time because they claim to have insomnia. They have to stop using these pills since they may become addicted to these pills soon.

You may now wonder if there are other ways to deal with stress, which do not include harming your body. Well, there definitely is and that way is using essential oils. You could use these oils to calm yourself and keep yourself happy and healthy. You will find yourself healthier if you use essential oils since these oils have multiple benefits.

Chronic Illness

If you are someone who has been suffering from certain illnesses like sinusitis or arthritis, you will have to consume the medicines that have been prescribed to you in order to keep the pain at bay. These drugs would have to be consumed regularly in order to ensure that the pain does not come back. These drugs may have adverse effects on your skin, which would mean that you would have to identify safer ways to help and heal yourself from the pain that would be through essential oils.

The essential oils have always worked well when used to heal the pain of the joints. You will have to massage certain essential oils on the joints to ensure that you do not have too much pain. You could also get rid of the headaches, the cold and also the aches around your temples when you inhale the smell of the essential oil. When you use essential oils, you will find that you can obtain benefits, which would ensure that you do not have any issues with your health in the future. There are a few essential oils that have been mentioned in the book that would help you learn which oil you can use in certain situations.

Chapter 3: Essential Oils for Healing

As mentioned above, essential oils have a lot of properties that make them essential and useful to the body. But, you have to ensure that you do not use more than what is necessary ever. Since these oils have always been extracted from natural substances, they have properties that would not be found in any chemically treated product. That being said, it is dangerous to consume too much of the oil since it is potent. In this chapter, you will learn the different ways by which you can consume the oils in order to heal yourself.

Inhalation of the oil

This is a technique that is used by most people since they will be able to obtain the properties of the essential oil directly. You will find that the oils have triggered the right response from you without any delay. There are different ways by which you can inhale the oil which are covered by this section.

Direct Inhalation

This is the simplest way by which one can obtain the properties of the essential oil. You can smell the essential oil easily when you are in the process of healing yourself.

Diffusion

This is another simple way by which you will be able to inhale the oils. The oils are converted to vapor, which then are inhaled by you. You will need to obtain the right type of diffuser since the type of the diffuser has a very strong effect on the constituency if the oil. Only when the consistency is right will the diffuser convert the oil into its right form of vapor.

Use a Humidifier

A person who has an issue with breathing will be able to use a humidifier in order to inhale the essential oils. You will need to buy the right type of a humidifier to which you will need to add the water. When the water is hot enough, you will have to pour a few drops of the essential oil onto a piece of tissue. This tissue will then have to be placed in front of the humidifier. This will trap the vapor of the oil into the humidifier, which would then be inhaled by you.

Steam

Take a large vessel and place it on the gas with water. Once the water has boiled, you will need to add a few drops of the essential oil into the vessel. You will then have to place your head over the vessel and cover your head and the vessel to ensure that the vapors do not escape from your face. You will need to constantly have to breathe in order to obtain the properties of the oil.

Application of the oil on certain body parts

When you purchase an essential oil, you will find a set of instructions at the back of the box that would help you learn how to apply the oil onto your body. It is best to dilute the essential with one of the carrier oils in order to ensure that you reduce the potency of the oil since the pure oil will be highly potent. You will need to ensure that you only apply the essential oil on the parts of the body that are mentioned below.

- The sole of your feet

- The temples behind the ears

- The forehead

- The crown of the head

- The neck

- The top of your ankle

There are a few techniques that you could use if you are trying to apply the essential oil on different parts of your body. These techniques are extremely simple are explained clearly in the section below.

Direct Application

The best way to apply essential oils to your skin is through direct application of the oil on your body. Take a drop of the oil and apply it on your body in a circular motion continuously. This would ensure that the oil is absorbed by your body.

Massage oil

The simplest and easiest way to make sure that the oil that you are applying on your body is absorbed by your body is by a massage. Take four drops of the essential oil on your palm and rub the oil across both your palms. Now, apply the oil on the part of your body and move your palms in a circular motion with a certain amount of pressure. Ensure that you use an essential oil that will not harm your skin at all.

If you find the oil too potent for your skin, you will need to add vegetable oil to the essential oil to create a blend that would then reduce the potency of the oil.

Oral Consumption

This is one of the best ways to consume certain essential oils. But, it is this very process that would leave you with danger since the essential oils are potent to an extent. You will find that your body has been affected in adverse ways if you do not take care of the quantity of the oil that you use. This section helps you understand the different ways by which you would be able to consume the essential oils orally.

Numerous scientists and medical experts have conducted research to understand the benefits of essential oils and also to identify how they can be consumed orally. You would have to ensure that you do not sip on the oils the way you would sip on wine or water. You will need to ensure that you have the purest form of the oil when it comes to oral consumption. You could also use these oils as dietary supplements. You would have to meet with your doctor to understand how much of the oil you will need to consume without causing yourself any harm. After that, you will need to read the instructions that have been given behind the essential oils bottle in order to ensure that you follow the right ways to consume oil.

- If you find it difficult to control the flow of the essential oil, you will need to consume a pill that would contain the essential oil. In order to neutralize the potency of the oil, you will need to neutralize it with water. You have to ensure that you drop the pill far back on your tongue and ensure that you wash it down with a lot of water!

- The other option would be to add three or four drops of the essential oil to a glass of milk.

- When you are cooking, you will need to ensure that you add a few drops of the essential oil to the pan. You could also use the oil when you are baking or making bread.

Tips on how to use essential oils responsibly

Essential oils in their pure form are often concentrated which makes them terribly dangerous to use without care. You will need to ensure that you can handle the potency of the essential oils depending on the part of the body you are going to use the oils. To ensure that you do this correctly, you will need to follow certain rules that have been explained clearly in the section below.

1. When you begin to use essential oils, you will have to ensure that you use a drop orifice to ensure that you are using the right proportion of the oil. You will know what the right proportion of the oil is when you approach your doctor to understand the same. When you have a child at home, you will need to ensure that you use a drop orifice since you have to ensure that your child is not affected adversely by the oil. If you find that either you or your child have consumed more than necessary, drink a glass of milk and rush to the doctor as fast as you can!

2. If you want to use the essential oil on your children, you have to ensure that you meet the doctor before you do use the oils. You have to ensure that there are no grave consequences to using the essential oils.

3. Right before you begin to use any essential oil, you have to ensure that the essential oil does not harm you in any way. You have to ensure that your skin does not react adversely to the oil. For this, you will need to test the oils on your skin to ensure that you are not allergic. You will need to ensure that your skin does not turn red or form a rash before you use the essential oils on any other part of your body. If there is any adverse reaction, you can use vegetable oil to neutralize the reaction or place your hand under cold water.

4. You should never use oils individually; it is always good to use them in the form of a blend. Before you use these blends, you will need to test them on certain parts of

your skin and wait to see if your skin reacts adversely to the oil.

5. There are some essential oils whose potency is very high that it affects an inanimate object and may affect your skin. You have to ensure that these oils do not come anywhere close to your contact lenses since you may be damaging them permanently. There is a possibility that you will harm your eyes too. If you have applied oil on your lenses, remove them immediately and wash them in cold water and vegetable oil.

6. You have to ensure that you do not apply any essential oils near your ears since that may prove to be fatal.

7. You have to identify the adverse effects of the essential oils on your skin when you are out in the sun.

8. Essential oils should never be used if you have used cosmetics. This is because of the fact that the essential oils begin to absorb the chemicals in the cosmetics and will send them into the blood stream. These chemicals then settle down in the fat tissues in your body.

If you have been injured recently and have any scars on your body, you will need to avoid using the oils on those very areas.

Chapter 4: Extraction of Essential Oils

You may already be aware of the fact that the essential oils are all extracted from the different parts of the plant. The oils have been used for multiple purposes and not only in aromatherapy. These oils have been found in many products like soaps, cosmetics, food, beverages and perfumes. There are certain processes of extraction, which have been mentioned in this chapter. There are traditional methods and there are modern methods, which have been known to give the best results. There is also a certain section at the end of the chapter that leaves you with two methods you could use to extract the essential oils from the leaves and flowers of the required herb.

It always depends on the type of oil you are looking for which would determines the plant that you must use in the extraction process. For some plants you use the flowers while for others you may use the leaves. There are other plants whose essential oils are extracted from the bark of the tree or the fruit. You will have to identify which part to use in order to obtain the purest form of the oil.

The different methods of extraction that have become popular have been mentioned below and the steps have been mentioned which would help you understand that there are no chemicals in the extraction of the oil.

Hydro distillation

This is a method that has become a very large industrial process and has been used to extract oil from the plants. There are three types of hydro distillation that have been perfected over the years – water distillation, water and steam distillation and direct steam distillation. The major difference between these types is the way the materials are handled during the process. The next part of this section explains to you how essential oils are extracted using this process.

What is Hydro distillation?

This is the most common type of method to extract essential oils from the leaves and flowers of the herbs in these modern times. There are three different methods to distill the flowers and leaves in this method but the common element of these methods is steam. The steam is what breaks the oil glands in the leaves and flowers and will help in releasing the oils from within the glands. You will need to put the leaves and the flowers into water and boil it in order to ensure that the oils are released from the tissues. This vapor is condensed and cooled in order to separate it from the water that can be done using a separator. This would involve three processes listed below.

-        The first process is hydro diffusion that involves the diffusion of the water and the oils from the membranes of the plants.

-        The next process if hydrolysis.

-        The last is the decomposition through heat.

Making an oil distiller at home

If you wish to use the hydro extractor method at home, then you will need a distiller for it. Distiller is a machine that you can use to extract the oil out from the raw materials. It is quite easy to make a distiller at home but if you don't want to make the effort then you can buy one.

They are easily available online and you can order one for yourself. They need not be too big and you can choose a medium or small sized distiller, as you will only be using it for your home use. The price of the distiller will vary depending on the size and the brand that you pick. A regular small oil distiller will cost you around $170 but you will only be able to extract a little oil at a time. A bigger one might cost you around $500.

However, you can build one at home by yourself. Here is what you will need for it.

- 1 pressure cooker
- 10 mm copper wire, 12 meters long
- 1 plastic tube, 2 inches long
- 1 bucket to large enough to hold coiled tube
- Good quality sealant
- Glass jar
- Mini sterilized bottles

You can buy the pressure cooker online. The size you pick will depend on how much oil you wish to extract.

To make the distiller, start by closing all the open valves on the lid of the cooker using the sealant. Leave just the steam valve free.

Once done, use the plastic tube to place over the steam valve. You should cover it fully at the bottom to secure it so that the steam directly moves into the plastic tube and not anywhere else.

Now use a cylinder or any cylindrical object to wrap the copper tube in the center and create a coil.

Your distiller is now ready to use. Here is how you can use it.

1. The first step is for you to gather all the raw ingredients that you will extract the oil from. This can include lavender flowers or orange peels etc. It is best to pick the best quality raw materials and give them a good wash.
2. Next, roughly chop the ingredients and add it to the pressure cooker vessel.
3. Add in enough water to cover the materials. Ensure that you use distilled water.
4. Next, fill the bucket with cold water. Some people add in ice but you can avoid the step if you think you will end up freezing the water. That will defeat the purpose of this particular activity!
5. Now tightly cover the lid on top and place the large tub on a stool next to the cooker.
6. Place the copper tube inside the bucket of water and the other end should be placed inside a collection jar.
7. Switch on the heat under the cooker.
8. Allow it to steam for 30 minutes to an hour or until you are satisfied with the amount of oil that is collected in the jar.
9. Once done, switch off the heat and wait for 5 minutes or until all the oil carrying liquid has been collected in the jar.
10. You can now wait for the liquid to cool down and you will see that the essential oil has floated to the top.
11. You can use a small dropper to extract the essential oil from top and place it in a sterilized bottle.
12. Add a label to the bottle and store it in a dark place for 24 to 48 hours in order to enhance its color and aroma.
13. You might also have to add the date in order to calculate the use by date.
14. Since it is quite concentrated, you will only need a small amount of it.

The distiller method works on a very simple scientific basis. As you know, pressure cookers create a pressure inside themselves that causes the water in it to convert to steam. This steam escapes from the steam valve that is present on the lid of the cooker. This steam mostly carries the flavor of whatever has been added inside the cooker.

So, when you add in the raw materials, the heat from the water causes its oils to release. That oil gets mixed with the water and converts to steam. That steam is then released through the valve into the tubing. When hot steam hits the cold copper tubing, it converts to water due to condensation. This water has the essential oil dissolved in it and is what gets collected in the final jar.

You can then easily collect the oil from top as oil is lighter than the water and it will float on top.

This is the same technique that many industries use to press the oil out. This technique will produce the purest oil that will be free from any impurities.

Notes:

Be sure to use a good quality pressure cooker and wash it immediately after pressing oil from one ingredient. Leaving the ingredient in for too long might cause it to leave behind stains and a strong smell that will interfere with your next press.

You can have different cookers to extract the different oils if you like. Although it will cost you a little extra, you will be able to avoid the colors and aromas from all getting mixed up.

You have to only use glass jars to both catch the oil+ water and also transfer the essential oil. Glass will not react with these whereas plastic will.

You must avoid exposing your essential oils to direct sun. Sunlight might cause its color and concentration to fade. Choose a dark room in advance to transport your essential oils safely.

The home extraction method is great as it will be cost effective.

Carbon dioxide extraction

This process is also called super critical fluid extraction that is a process of extracting solvents from the leaves and flowers. Carbon dioxide is kept under extreme pressure that would turn it into its liquid form. The liquid works as a solvent to extract the oils from the leaves and the flowers by diffusing through the. The final products of the process will generally be the same but this cannot be said about every type of oil.

The best part about using this method is that the aroma of the oil will remain strong and fragrant and will resemble the fragrance of the plant! This process does have its disadvantages too. You would need to invest a lot of time and money into this process, which may or may not be feasible. This is due to the fact that the equipment is expensive and there could be residues of certain fertilizers and pesticides in the plant products, which may hinder the process. You would also have to conduct a lot of research before you invest yourself in this process.

Solvent extraction

You may have gathered that you do not have the chance to use the fragile parts of a plant when it comes to extracting oil from them. This process uses certain solvents like ethanol, ether, petroleum ether, methanol and hexane. These solvents are required to extract certain lipophilic materials from the parts of the plant. The extract from this process would generally be thick since the tissue of the plant and the chlorophyll is also extracted. This is the first product that is called the concrete. This product is now added to undenatured alcohol that would then give the complete product that is called the absolute.

The final product has a very low residue but there are certain aroma therapists who have said that the product may have certain pesticides in them. These would result in negative effects that may not relieve you from your pain. This product is heavily concentrated and has the fragrance of the plant. It is because of this reason that these products are used to prepare perfumes.

There are many other modern techniques like micro distillation, thermos – micro distillation, microwave distillation and protoplast distillation which have come into view over the last few years. None of these methods use any chemical, which ensures that the essential oils are in their purest forms and would never cause you any harm.

DIY Extraction of essential oils

As promised above, this section contains the two methods that will help you make essential oil at home! You will find these methods very simple and easy to execute!

Extraction of oils using oil

You may think this is a very surprising thing to do. How would one be able to extract an essential oil using another form of oil? This section leaves you with the method you could use to extract the oil. This process works on the principle of the law of attraction – oil attracts oil. You will be able to extract the oils from the flowers and the leaves of the plant by soaking them in oil.

1. You must first take a container, preferably nonmetal and add the required amount of olive oil to the

container. You will need to add the leaves and the flowers of the plant whose oil you would like to extract.

2. Cover the container well with a nonmetal lid and leave it aside for a couple of days.

3. Begin to strain the mixture of the herbs and the oil by pressing the flowers and the leaves together gently. You will be able to release more quantity of oil when you do this.

4. Then add a few extra leaves and flowers to the container and follow the same steps as mentioned above.

5. You may have to perform these steps repeatedly in order to obtain a rich form of the essential oil!

6. Store the essential oil in a dark place and in a vial that is airtight and is sealed well.

How to extract oils by using alcohol

This method is very simple and is completely fool proof. You will first need to soak the flowers and the leaves of the plant whose oil you want to extract in alcohol. You have to ensure that the alcohol that you use is undenatured ethyl alcohol. If you are unable to find the undenatured alcohol, you could use alcohol but bear in mind that you must never use rubbing alcohol.

The next few steps that you will need to follow are the same as the steps that have been mentioned above. If you want, you could use pure alcohol or you could use a diluted version of the alcohol. You could use alcohol since you could end up using the oil as a perfume! This will save you the trouble of looking for the best perfume out there!

When you decide to separate the oil from the alcohol or the water, you will have to leave the container in the blast freezer. When this is done, you will find that the oil has coagulated at the top of the container. Since this oil does not freeze, you will be able to scrape the oil off with ease. This is a process that you could use when you are using delicate flowers in order to avoid marring the flowers and the leaves.

Chapter 5: Essential Oils and Their Health Benefits

The first few chapters explained to you about aromatherapy and essential oils. You have also been given an idea on what the advantages of using essential oils are. You now have to have an idea on what the health benefits of the essential oils are. When you complete this chapter, you will know which essential oil you will need to use!

Lavender oil

Lavender oil is something that can become every person's best friend! It plays an extremely important role in the lines of caring for your skin. You will be able to treat any form of acne, scars or spots when you use this oil. The oil can be used to cleanse your skin and also help in returning it to its original complexion. You will find that the oil can be used when it comes to releasing any anxiety, stress or fatigue.

Neroli oil

This oil has multiple properties – an aphrodisiac, antiseptic and an anti – depressant. It has often been used to treat the skin and clear it of any blemishes that may have been caused by spots or scars. You will also be able to get rid of any gas that may be inside your body based on the application of the oil. The next chapter gives you the different ways by which you can use this oil!

Lemon oil

A person with oily skin will find this oil good for them since the oil has a property of an astringent that would help in improving their complexion and skin quality.

Rose oil

Rose oil is also an astringent but has the added benefit of being an anti – depressant. These two properties of the oil help in improving the mental health of a person thereby improving the physical health of the person.

Tea Tree oil

This oil is great to fight off any type of diseases. You will find that the oil can be used to remove any kind of smell or any fungal infection. You will also be able to remove any form of acne and blemish on your skin.

Sandalwood oil

Sandalwood oil has always played an important role when it has come to skin care. You will find that the oil has properties which help in repairing damaged skin and turning it into healthy looking skin in no time. You will find the scars vanishing from your face in no time. This oil has also been used to relieve people of any form of stress that they may be in. The most important use of this oil is that it has been used in numerous perfumes since the oil has an extremely strong fragrance.

Pine oil

Pine oil is the best antimicrobial agent. It is also often used as a stimulant when it comes to healing stress and anxiety. You will also be able to use the oil in different perfumes in order to calm your nerves.

Geranium oil

A person with acne and oily skin will consider geranium oil to be their best friend. The oil also has a property that helps in the tightening of skin, which helps in reducing the wrinkles on your skin as you grow. The oil also has healing properties that help in treating burns and bruises.

Eucalyptus oil

Eucalyptus oil has often been known for its fragrance that has always been overpowering. It also has a flavor that is unique to it and gives it the properties of a repellant or an antiseptic. The oil is known to improve the immunity of the body when the oil is used regularly. You will also be able to avoid any headaches that you often have and the common cold!

Clove oil

Clove oil is probably the best oil that a person with dry skin can use! The oil is known for the properties that make the oil a worthy sedative. Let us assume that you have a toothache. You could apply a drop of the oil onto your tooth that would help in creating a smooth flow of blood and also help in relieving you of the pain. You will find that the oil also helps in the increase of the levels of energy.

These are a few of the benefits of the commonly used essential oils.

Chapter 6: Essential Oils to Keep You Healthy

This chapter covers the essential oils that you can use to keep yourself healthy. You will also be able to lose weight. Essential oils have been proven to help in weight loss too. It is known to help curb your hunger pangs. There are certain essential oils that help in losing weight. There are quite a few factors that help in reducing weight. You will find that the different properties of the oils mentioned below will aid in your chance to lose weight.

Cinnamon oil

This oil is often extracted from the bark if the tree called the cinnamomum tree. You will also be able to obtain the oil from the leaves of the plant. You will find that the level of sugar in your blood is easily controlled when you use this essential oil. You will find yourself losing the weight that you have gained due to lack of resistance of insulin. When you use this oil you will find that the insulin levels have been regulated which helps in boosting your immune system too. The blood starts to circulate well in your body and also helps in clearing your intestines.

Fennel oil

The oil is obtained from seeds that have been distilled in steam. This oil helps you in improving your digestion and also in curbing your pangs of hunger. You will also be able to have a good amount of sleep!

Grapefruit Oil

This oil has often been used as an antiseptic by the doctors in the ancient days. It was also used as a disinfectant and helps in getting rid of any excess water that your body may have retained. You will also find that this oil helps in curbing any pangs of hunger that you may feel during the day. The added advantage of this oil is that it helps you get rid of the excess fat that is found in your abdomen since it has a compound calling Nootaktone that is known to absorb any extra fat. You could consume a few drops of the oil mixed in a glass of water, which would help you lose weight with ease.

Lemongrass oil

This oil is extracted from the stalk of the plant. This oil helps you in clearing your skin of acne and also helps in reducing your excess body weight. You will also find yourself being relieved of any pains or aches.

Lemon oil

The lemon oil is obtained by cold pressing the peels of the lemon. This oil is great at helping you avoid gaining any weight. This oil also helps in enhancing your mood and also helps in relieving any pain you may feel. You will find yourself with increased levels of energy and a better rate of metabolism, which helps in the release of toxins from your body. The other advantage of this oil is that the parasites in the intestines are killed which saves you from any digestive problems. You will find that the smell of this oil is enough to help you lose weight and keep digestive problems at bay.

Spearmint oil

This oil is a great help when it comes to keeping your digestive system clean. It helps in speeding up the process and also helps in reducing bloating. The oil has the power to calm your muscles down which ensures that you do not feel hungry too often. You will find yourself with immense energy and will also be able to stay alert. The added advantage is that the oil helps in curing the common cold and a fever! How great is it that you can strike three birds with just one type of oil?

Peppermint oil

This oil has properties that are similar to that of the spearmint oil. It aids in digestion and also helps in reducing bloating. The oil has tons of nutrients that are beneficial to your body. When you inhale this oil, you will find yourself less hungry than you were a few seconds ago. It is always good to inhale this oil since the oil will be able to run its magic faster than you can say Essential Oils. There is a possibility that this oil may be too strong to inhale. At such a time you will have to consume the oil orally in the form of a solution. Since inhaling this oil will help in curbing your appetite, you could use the oil in your bath!

Chapter 7: Essential Oils and Stress Relief

A lot of research has been conducted to understand why people are under stress. It was found that 92% of the people always approach their doctors with a complaint that they have been suffering headaches that are unbearable. This is because of the fact that they have chronic stress. You have to remember that there are quite a few diseases that could be caused due to chronic stress of which strokes are the most common. You will find that you have a higher chance of dying at a younger age when compared to any other disease. You will also find yourself stressing about the wrong reasons since your brain perceives that you are under stress irrespective of whether or not you literally are. It is always because of this that you will find yourself stressed. You will then start worrying about the stress and find yourself under more stress. This is when you will begin to find yourself getting stressed immensely.

A person who is found with chronic stress has been treated with essential oils. This is the treatment that has become very common these last few years all across the world. The essential oils have certain components in them that help in spreading a sense of calm and relief throughout your body. These oils undertake the role that they are required of – they could work towards producing a sense of calm or stimulate what the person is feeling. For example, if you administer one of the essential to a person who is not very confident of himself, the oil could work towards instilling a sense of confidence while if it were administered to a person who is under immense stress, he or she would find himself calming down. This is what gives them the name adaptogens since they change their role depending on what the person whom it is administered on is feeling.

This section covers a few oils that you could use when you are trying to relieve yourself of any stress that you may have been feeling due to the pressures of the day. These are the oils that are used most often when compared to the other essential oils.

Lavender oil

This oil is one of the few oils, which has a property, which rightly gives it the name Adaptogen. There were many studies that were conducted over the years that have proved that the people using this oil have appeared to be very calm and relaxed when compared with the people who did not. This study also proved that people who used this oil were always able to work out mathematical and financial equations with ease that showed that they were very alert.

Cedarwood oil

Cedarwood has been known across the world as a plant with numerous medicinal properties. It has been shown to give children suffering from ADHD and ADD certain amount of relief that helps in keeping them calm and at ease. This is because of the fact that this oil is known to help people calm their minds down within no time. You will find yourself releasing every bit of stress that you may have when you apply this oil on the stem of your brain.

Chamomile oil

A person with a short temper would do well to use chamomile oil. This is the one oil that helps in clearing your mind of any excessive stress that you may have and also helps in clearing your emotions within a few seconds. If you are someone who has too much stress, you will find that you are calm as a feather when you use this oil. You will also be able to rid yourself of the changing emotions that you have because of the stress. You will also be able to overcome any stressful situations without worrying about how you may react.

Jasmine oil

If you are someone who is often stressed about yourself and your confidence, you will find jasmine oil to be your best friend. When you use this oil, you will be able to find yourself optimistic at all times. You can use this oil when you find yourself depressed at any point in your life. This oil will also help you overcome and stress and insomnia too!

Chapter 8: Combinations of Oils to Use to Keep Yourself Happy!

The recipes that have been mentioned in this chapter leave you without any stress and keep you healthy. It is because of this that you find yourself happier than you ever were.

Anti-Cellulite Balm
Ingredients

- ☐ 5 drops cypress oil
- ☐ 5 drops ginger oil
- ☐ 25 drops grapefruit oil
- ☐ 5 drops peppermint oil
- ☐ 10 drops rosemary oil
- ☐ 1 tablespoon almond oil at every use

Method

1. Take a transparent vial and ensure that it is clean. Add the oils in the order mentioned above and fasten the vial.
2. Shake the ingredients well to ensure that they mix.
3. Store the vial in a dark and cold place that would ensure that the oils blend well.
4. You could apply two or three drops of oil on your body to reduce the fat in that area.

Belly Busting massage oil
Ingredients

- ☐ 10 drops cypress oil
- ☐ 10 drops grapefruit oil

- ☐ 10 drops juniper berry oil
- ☐ 5 drops sage oil
- ☐ 10 drops sweet orange oil
- ☐ 2 ounces almond oil

Method

1. Take a transparent vial and ensure that it is clean. Add the oils in the order mentioned above and fasten the vial.
2. Shake the ingredients well to ensure that they mix.
3. Store the vial in a dark and cold place that would ensure that the oils blend well.
4. Shake the oils well before you use it and warm two or three spoons of the oil and massage the oil well on your belly.

Aromatherapy anti stress massage oil

Ingredients

- ☐ 10 drops lavender oil
- ☐ 10 drops lemon oil
- ☐ 30 drops sage oil
- ☐ 5 ounces sweet almond oil or jojoba oil

Method

1. Take a transparent vial and ensure that it is clean. Add the oils in the order mentioned above and fasten the vial.
2. Shake the ingredients well to ensure that they mix.
3. Store the vial in a dark and cold place, which would ensure that the oils blend well.
4. You can always use this oil when you are going to sleep or if you have come back from work.

Aromatherapy Bath Salt
Ingredients

- ☐ 3 cups sea salt or Himalayan pink salt or Epsom salt
- ☐ 5 drops lavender oil
- ☐ 10 drops sandalwood oil
- ☐ 1 tablespoon jojoba oil

Method

1. Take a glass bowl and ensure that it is clean. Add the oils in the order mentioned above and fasten the vial.
2. Shake the ingredients well to ensure that they mix.
3. Move the mixture to a transparent vial.
4. You could add a tablespoon of this salt when you are filling your tub with water. You will need to mix the salt well. You will find yourself calm and stress free when you come out of the bath.

Conclusion

Thank you once again for purchasing the book.

This book contains all the information that you would need to know about aromatherapy and also the essential oils that you would need to use for aromatherapy. These oils have multiple benefits that have been listed out in the book. But, before you gather information into all that you would have to learn what aromatherapy is which has been mentioned to you explicitly in the first chapter of the book. The latter chapters of the book give you details on how you will need to take care of yourself using the essential oils. Thank you once again. I hope you have gathered all the information that you were looking for.